SILENT ANGER

SILENT ANGER

Danny E. Blanchard, PhD. P.C.

Library of Congress Control Number:		2018901031
ISBN:	Hardcover	978-1-5434-8062-7
	Softcover	978-1-5434-8061-0
	eBook	978-1-5434-8060-3

Print information available on the last page.

Rev. date: 02/06/2018

To order additional copies of this book, contact:
Xlibris
1-888-795-4274
www.Xlibris.com
Orders@Xlibris.com
772711

TABLE OF CONTENTS

DEDICATION

This book is dedicated to a woman of God who has always put her family above everything. A mother of 9 children, 22 grandchildren, 23 great-grandchildren, and 2 great-great grandchildren. Your love and care will always be remembered. With this in mind, this book is dedicated with the highest respect and love to

Thomy Dale Burnett

ACKNOWLEDGEMENTS

Many family members, professional colleagues, and researchers assisted me with my latest book publication.

Dr. Mildred Johnson who always served as a positive motivator, and constantly encouraging me to complete my research. Ms. Lovey Verdun, former registrar at Oakwood University in Huntsville, Alabama. She always displayed kindness and concern about my research.

Dr. Raymond Winbush, Dr. Earl Gooding, Dr. Barry Black and Dr. Mervyn Warren Sr. are individuals who have been an inspiration and motivation in dealing with the ills of our society. Their ideas, concepts and theories assisted me with the overall research and design of my book.

Mrs. Deanja M. Nelson my typist, who provided excellent clerical work with the manuscript. Mrs. Shalonda White who designed the book jacket, with her excellent artistry and color scheme.

Mrs. Chammand Deesnit who assisted with the designing of the short stories. They brought a great deal of life to the history of Mental-Health in America.

Ms. Carol Ward for invaluable clerical support and the editing of each draft.

Finally, I must thank Dr. Lola Brown for her love, motivation, and respect throughout the research of this book.

Danny E. Blanchard PhD., P.C.

SILENT ANGER

Let us look at this peculiar institution known as Slavery and
its impact on the Mental Health of African-Americans.

"The Beginning"

Danny E. Blanchard, PhD. P.C.

Dr. Danny E. Blanchard is a former university professor with over *25* years of experience in dealing with mental health care in African Americans and Mexican Americans. He is the recipient of numerous local academic and state awards.

Dr. Blanchard has served on numerous mental health boards and has served as a mental health state advisor to the former Governor of the State of Alabama, Governor Don Siegleman.

Dr. Blanchard is a much sought-after speaker and consultant in various areas concerning mental health care. He is board certified in Mental Health Counseling, and Marriage and Family Therapy and is currently in private practice, which he has been for *25* years.

Dr. Blanchard is the author of two widely read books, Black Men Do Cry and Well Water, The Psychological Effects of Racism on African American Children.

Dr. Blanchard is a graduate of Oakwood University with a degree in psychology and he holds advance degrees from Loma Linda University, in Loma Linda, California, and in Vanderbilt University in Nashville, TN. He has done additional graduate studies at the University of California, Riverside Campus, Riverside, California.

Dr. Blanchard has a strong commitment to the mental health care of all people, both in the United States and abroad. He has had the opportunity to assist people with individual mental health needs from all cultures and ethnic groups.

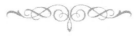

He has a strong belief that mental health care should be America's number one health concern, and has dedicated his life to seeing to it that all people are cared for in regard to their mental health needs.

It is the hope that the readers of this book will gain additional insight into the mental health needs of America's people of color; and more specifically, all people.

SILENT ANGER

Mental health in the African-American community has never fully been studied historically considering the impact of Slavery. When we consider this relationship between Mental health and Slavery, questions begin to arise. How is Slavery characterized? Was slavery a disease? Or, was it simply a means for economic gain that incidentally resulted in the desecration of a culture due to greed manifested within slave traders and profiteers?

There is no doubt that it is important to understand the impact that Slavery had on the mental health of those who were impacted by this institution.

Join me as we explore how Slavery created the most hideous mental health problems that African-Americans have experienced, and continue to experience in American society today.

SILENT ANGER

A History of Mental Health Care in Black America.

There was little advancement in mental health care, and what little was known was surely not available to slaves. Slaves were not placed in clinical therapy or psychiatric attention. Nor were they given adequate medical support.

Slaves were never given treatment for psychosis, neurosis, depression, stress, anxiety, or any mental health related issues. The only treatment given for such conditions were beatings, lashes, or inhumane tactics to solicit obedience from the disabled slave.

Danny E. Blanchard, PhD. PC.

SILENT ANGER

Slave owners believed that teaching a slave to hate himself
was far worse and more criminal than to teach him to hate
someone else.

Danny E. Blanchard, PhD. P.C

SILENT ANGER

Mental health issues grew rampant during the years of
Slavery. Black Americans did not passively develop mental
and behavioral limitations. They were taken from well-
structured, organized, healthy environments in various
parts of Africa. They did not come to America depressed,
psychotic, neurotic, suicidal, or bi-polar. They developed
these disorders as a result of being captured and brought to
America as slaves.

Slaves left a culture, religion, family, economic, social,
educational, and financial system, and a healthy lifestyle of
their own. Slaves spoke their own language and all had no
interest in learning their slave masters language and culture,
once brought to America.

Danny E. Blanchard, PhD. P.C

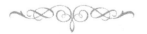

SILENT ANGER

During the Civil War, many African-Americans fought on the side of the confederacy because they feared that the Union Army would make their lives even more intolerable. Despite having the support of black soldiers, many felt that they could only be used as maintenance workers: latrine duty, cooks, maids, road maintenance, and those who were assigned to laundry details of the confederate soldiers.

The fact that slaves could neither read or write made it far more difficult for them to function independent of white confederate officers. Moreover, superstition and fear of being reprimanded discouraged many slaves from abandoning the institutions of their slave owners and instead, led them to fight for survival in the confederate unit and uniform.

Danny E. Blanchard, PhD. P.C

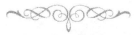

SILENT ANGER

Mental Health Care in the African-American Community

Danny E. Blanchard, PhD. P.C

INTRODUCTION

Good mental health is essential to every human being, and lack of it can cause sickness in any part of the body. Everyone experiences emotional roller coasters throughout their lives, however, how we handle these emotions matter. Mental health transcends our emotions to affect our way of thinking and our reactions; it can change lives and relationships with the people around us and can affect anyone. However, with proper treatment, one can still live a relatively normal, healthy life. In this book, I will specifically address mental health in the African American society. I shall discuss the causes of mental health problems, prevalence, outcomes and reasons why many African-American resist seeking treatment and services.

Prevalence

Despite the fact that anyone can develop a mental health problem, the African- American community seems to be most affected compared to the rest of the population in the United States of America. Statistics show that more African-Americans experience feelings of sadness, desperation, and triviality than whites. Moreover, further research shows that 8.2% of the African-American teenagers attempted suicide as compared to 6.2% of white teenagers.

Causes of Mental Health Problems in the African-American Community: Racism and Slavery

Long periods of slavery and discrimination of African-Americans continue to have an impact on their social and economic status. Slavery and racial discrimination are two major conventions that have largely contributed to the socioeconomic disparities that they experience. These have led to exclusion from proper health, educational, social and economic resources. Despite the vast strides made over the years regarding racial discrimination, it continues to negatively impact the mental health of African Americans. Negative stereotypes and rejection continue to occur, bringing with them undesirable consequences such as the mistrust of authorities who appear to not be in their favor. Many are exposed to violence and trauma-related situations where a broader community is assigned to fight in the military.

Homelessness

Homelessness has been considered a factor that contributes to mental health problems among African Americans. A study revealed that those who suffer from mental health complications comprise over 40% of the entire homeless population in the Unites States. Therefore, those who experience homelessness are at a higher risk of developing mental health issues. Furthermore, the homeless and runaway youth tend to suffer from mental health conditions at shockingly high rates.

Foster Care and Child Welfare Services

A significant number of children placed in the public foster care system comprise of African Americans with almost half of those kids awaiting adoption (Young, Griffith & Williams, 2013). These children are often victims of abuse or neglect. In that order, they are frequently moved from one home to another. Such conditions places them at a higher risk to develop poor mental health conditions. According to an epidemiological research, forty-two percent of the children and teenagers in the welfare system reported having met the DSM-V criteria for mental disorder.

Exposure to Violence

African-American children have been recorded to have a higher probability of being exposed to violence than other children. While some are victims of physical abuse, others know someone who has suffered violence. This has led to increased risks of developing mental disorders such as depression, anxiety, and post-traumatic disorders.

Reasons Why African-Americans do not Seek Treatment

Contrary to the research showing that many African Americans are victims of mental disorders, further research shows that many of those affected do not seek medical treatment at all. Others fail to finish their treatment or follow up. Some of these reasons for failure to seek treatment include:

Ignorance and Misunderstanding

In the African-American community, many perceive psychiatric disorders as a form of punishment from God or personal weakness. Therefore, it is widely assumed that it is something that someone just needs to 'snap out of'. A result of this mentality is that many shy away from treatment because fear of stigmatization or ridicule.

Faith, Spirituality, and Community

Family, society, and religion have been an excellent source of strength and support for African• Americans throughout history. Therefore, when experiencing mental health complications, they are more likely to turn to their families, communities or religion for help instead of seeking professional advice. While family or religious influences can provide some solution or give comfort, some situations may be too severe, and professional medical treatment must be sought.

Inaccessibility and Reluctance to Seek Mental Health Services

While some might not be able to access health services, many are reluctant to use psychological health services. Reasons for their reluctance may include: lack of trust for the health caregiver or fear of misdiagnosis. Over the years, African Americans have experience first-hand discrimination and prejudice, and the lack of cultural competence by health professionals make many African-Americans shy away from treatment.

Common Mental Health Conditions

Depression

There is more into depressive disorder than just feeling sad and hopeless. Such a condition could have severe consequences for both the victim and those around him or her. Therefore, early diagnosis and treatment is required. While some might experience depression only once in their lifetime, for others it becomes a recurring experience. It is characterized by changes in sleep, loss of appetite, experiencing suicidal thoughts, lack of concentration, and feelings of guilt, despair, and sadness.

Attention Deficit Hyperactivity Disorder

This condition is characterized by hyperactivity. It is mostly diagnosed in children who are between the ages of 3-17, however, some adults may also share this diagnosis. Most of the time the victim becomes easily distracted, jumps from one activity to another, and has trouble completing tasks. The victim may appear to be very careless and loses items easily, always daydreaming and has a difficult time paying attention.

Suicide

A high number of youth compared to adults often commit suicide. Suicidal thoughts are severe and require immediate attention from a professional. Usually, a person who can be termed as ruinous portray the following signs: frequently talks about taking their lives, extremely aggressive, socially withdrawn, experience suicidal thoughts and have unpredictable mood swings.

Posttraumatic Stress Disorder (PTSD)

Many African-Americans who have been victims of violence and abuse have PTSD. Therefore, there is a need for immediate treatment and therapy to avoid any adverse consequences. It is mainly characterized by intrusive memories that often reveal the traumatic episode, keeping a distance from certain places and objects, having out-of-body experiences, regular anger outbursts, and being startled easily.

Treatment of the Mental Disorder

Once realizing that you or your loved one suffers from a psychiatric illness, it is essential that one seeks professional assistance to help prevent any further damage. Studies show that many African• Americans who have tried treatment and completed the treatment requirements have demonstrated significant improvement in their health and lifestyle (Logan, Denby & Gibson, 2013). The Affordable Care Act has been put in place to ensure that they can be able to access affordable treatment for their conditions. Treatments for mental health conditions include psychotherapy and support groups, medications such as antidepressants and antipsychotics along with brain stimulation therapies. All these are provided to assist the individual in the process of healing and facilitates their transition to living a healthy life. Also, after treatments, follow-ups are made to ensure and document progress.

Conclusion

Many African-Americans are faced with other challenges in addition to their social and economic conditions. Due to their beliefs, culture, and

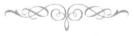

religion, many of them seek alternative medical treatment. Some of the choices of treatment may work well while some may not bring out the desired outcome.

Some fear medical therapies due to biased medical professionals and racists who might give misdiagnosis. However, instead of avoiding getting treatment at all, it is advisable for one to find a health care provider who suits their needs.

SILENT ANGER

The degree to which black American slaves were subjected to Mental Health cruelty is remarkable.

For over 400 years, slaves in America were given poor food substance, insufficient healthcare, and placed to live under inhumane living conditions. Prenatal care was not provided by slave owners. Many slave children were born with severe mental disorders, attention deficit disorders, and mental retardation. Hydrocephalic and micro cephalic brain disorders were common and many children were underweight.

Many pregnant slaves, who worked long hours on slave plantations, gave birth to babies that were stillborn, or babies who did not live very long. This was a result of the poor quality of prenatal care or the complete absence of prenatal care on the plantation.

Despite the pain and sorrow suffered, slave mothers would
often kill their babies, rather than have them placed in
Slavery.

Danny E. Blanchard, PhD. P.C

SILENT ANGER

We will begin with stories. Though they are fictitious, they will help to develop an understanding of what African-Americans must have experienced during the peculiar institution of Slavery.

Danny E. Blanchard, PhD. P.C.

Physical, Emotional and Sexual Abuse on the Plantation

'Too sweet', how they called her, was a young girl. At a delicate age, like many children in her time, she had fallen victim to slavery for the purpose of sexual exploitation.

Her innocent life changed suddenly around the age of twelve during puberty. Young men began to gape at her while she worked on the plantation and eventually her beauty became more apparent and caught the attention of her master.

One night a horrible incident occurred in her life that she would never ever forget. She was torn away from her mother's arms in the middle of the night.

"Mom, help me! Dad, help me!" Too Sweet screamed aloud.

Her parents were horrified to hear the loud cry of their beloved daughter. With frightened expressions on their faces, they looked around in the darkness and saw blurred figures around them.

"Be quiet or you all are dead!" uttered a voice. Instantly they recognized the voice was from their master.

In the darkness five men were standing in their primitive barrack. They threw her body on the ground and tore her night gown from her body. Her parents could not help her, because they were beaten up and shackled.

Before their eyes they were forced to watch their master and four other white men rape their daughter. After that horrible incident, they came again, pounding open the door every single night, just to satisfy their beastly passions. When Too Sweet was not willing to do what they wanted,

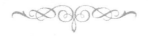

her mother and father were brutally beaten and tortured until she willingly gave her body to be humiliated.

Her parents cried while watching their little daughter plead for help. Their inability to help her broke their hearts in ways that were unimaginable.

"Lord have mercy!" Her mother screamed painfully while Too Sweet was crying and bearing the pain inflicted by her abusers. With great sorrow, her father looked at her and struggled to breathe.

"I am so sorry, Too Sweet, forgive me for not being able to protect you!" He cried as tears stained his face.

Too Sweet cried until there were no tears left to cry and the pain became numb. Helpless she let them do whatever they wanted to do with her.

Eventually, her father, no longer able to withstand the mental torment, took his own life. They found his body hanging from a tree. Next, her mother was brutally beaten and died from her injuries. Finally, Too Sweet was left alone and abandoned all hope. She was sold and forced into prostitution from plantation to plantation.

Children who were born as slaves had no right to be children, no right to express themselves, and especially young girls at that time, like Too Sweet, were forced into slavery. This led to numerous unwanted pregnancies and abortions which caused mental and physical mutilations, and sexually transmitted diseases.

It was an indignity for Too Sweet to be raped in front of her parents. She felt worthless and could not understand her purpose for existence as a slave.

Since her father's suicide and her mother's death, she no longer cared about her life. She could not even remember how many men she had been with. It was horrible that words could never describe how she, like the

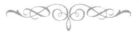

other victims, must have felt, but she knew that one day, the torture endure would end.

"Why could my life not be like the others, just because of my colored skin?" She thought.

This question remained in her mind until the day she suddenly fell very ill and her body became weak. Each day her condition became worse until she could not walk anymore. She had contracted syphilis.

No one cared about her and she was left sick and alone somewhere on a plantation, without food and water. At this point in her life she knew she would not have any chance of survival; she would surely die. With her last few breathes she uttered,

"This is my deliverance, Jesus, redeem me."

"Free me from this evil, Lord."

A day later, it would have been her fifteenth birthday, but sadly it was not to be. She was finally at peace.

"Loaded Sam the Fighter"

Loaded Sam was the master's main slave who was sent from plantation to plantation to fight other slaves until death, or until their bodies were ripped apart. Loaded Sam killed over 30 slaves in fights that rewarded him favor with his master. After each fight Sam would receive a large beer and a chicken. Sometimes the master would give Sam women to use for a week of drinking and womanizing on the plantation. In the end, Sam died of a heart attack after over 300 fights on various plantations.

Fear and intimidation on the plantation was a normal way of life for slaves, and all slaves suffered some type of mental and/or physical illness. Mental health issues were considered a normal part of life for even the children.

Depression, anxiety, suicide, fear, paranoia, psychosis, neurosis and bipolar illness were all a part of the slave behavior and at times were looked upon as a normal way of living. Slave masters wanted their slaves to be abnormal and mentally disturbed.

Slaves were not permitted to learn how to read, write, nor look at words. Slaves were constantly insulted, humiliated and degraded. They were required to act like animals and perform like circus clowns around the plantation.

Despite such heinous living arrangements, slaves enjoyed the company of one another primarily at night and in the fields. There they could discuss the issues of the day like who was sold, beaten, died, ran away or had a child.

Fear and evil acts toward slaves made their mental conditions much worse than one could imagine. Research has not even begun to provide a full

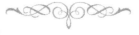

understanding to society as to the mental conditions that slaves were subjected to during that period.

The slave plantation was not really a plantation, it was a hole full of evil vice, hate, and using slaves as weapons to project their evil ways.

Danny E. Blanchard, PhD. P.C.

Prenatal Disorders on the Plantation

"Slow John! Feed the horses!" Yelled a man as he stared angrily at a little boy.

"And the horse dungs, boy! Don't forget everything that I am saying to you!" He added.

The little boy had no other choice but to obey. He followed and did what they told him to do. He was their slave.

He collected the horse dungs and placed them in a certain place beside a tent, leaving them to dry in the burning sun until they were capable of being used as fuel. Despite all his hard work, it was never good enough for his master. They exploited him and 'sucked' every ounce of energy from that little boy.

Like every slave, he had to follow his master's commands and was never allowed to express any word of disagreement or else he would be punished. The boy nodded to every order, and walking with a bent• over position he went to do as he was bidden by his master. Confusion was almost always laced in his expressions because he never understood why he had to do what they said. In fact, he was too little to understand why they treated him like this, with total disregard for his disability.

At the end of the long, hard work days, the only thing he would hear from his master were words spoken in anger.

"A sound thrashing has never done you no harm boy?" These words echoed in the ears of the little boy as his master's mischievous laugh filled the air.

The boy nodded in response still with a look of confusion upon his face. When the day was finally completed he would return to the lonely barn for rest.

In the loneliness of the night memories of his past flashed through his mind. Once he tried not to do what they said, but it only resulted in them tying him to a tree, shackling him, and leaving him days and nights in the wind and rain without food. After this treatment he would be set free and thrown into the barn that housed the horses who, in time, became his only friends.

When he was younger his former master sold him to a travelling circus because of his mental disability. His disability was as a result of his mother being raped and brutally beat during pregnancy. The birthing process was a difficult one and was very slow. It took a few days from the birth pangs until he saw the light of the day. Then they gave him the name 'Slow John'.

His master would have given him up without cost just to get rid of this burden, but for a little money, the circus director bought Slow John.

"I can use him for everything," thought the circus director while taking a look at the little boy. He motioned for the boy to follow him after the bargain was complete.

"Now, I am your master. You hear me boy? You listen to me now!" said the slave master as Slow John followed behind him.

In the travelling circus, they moved from town to town with animals, mostly horses, building their tents at far-off places, somewhere at the fringes of the town where they stopped.

The boy did whatever they wanted him to do whenever they wanted him to do it. To eat, Slow John salvaged the leftover food that he could find from the plates. He was fighting to survive, but it was not enough for him. He began to suffer from malnutrition and eventually he became extremely weak as his health worsened. No one cared about him and that little boy was left to starve.

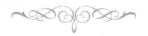

In the barn the boy knelt before his only friend, a white horse and as his body began to sink onto the ground, he stared into the eyes of the horse and began to speak.

"You are so beautiful, my friend!" The horse nodded in response and the boy continued.

"Don't forget me, my friend. I guess, I am called by the Lord today!" He struggled to bring a smile to his lips.

He was in a terrible state of exhaustion from starving and it was evident from the way his skin dung to his bones. His neck was bowed, his face and cheeks were thin, pale and emaciated. His eyes were sunken deep within their sockets. A face which normally should have been filled with cheerfulness as every child at the age of nine should be, he was scared with sorrow. His life was not like other children. He had always been a slave.

"I will see my mom soon." He said in a silent whisper.

Slowly, the light began to fade form his eyes as he settled in a patch of hay on the floor. He looked up and uttered his last words, "I am ready Lord!"

The next day his lifeless body was found on the floor before the horse. The horse stayed awake the whole night, watching over him. The soul of this little boy finally left his body. Though he died of hunger, he was now resting in peace.

Suicide on the Plantation-
"Moon Watcher"

The frail body of a mature man stood in the middle of a dark gloomy room with tears running down his bruised cheeks. He was staring at a rope that hung from the wooden beam above a nearby chair.

Bitterly he whispered, "They can take my body, but not my dignity", and began pressing his lips together.

He was called 'Moon Watcher'.

For a brief moment, he closed his eyes trying to recall a memory from his childhood. As a little boy, one night after the sun had gone to rest and the moon appeared like a pearl in the inky sky, his father looked up and asked,

"Do you see the moon son?" pulling his son close to him.

Lowering his voice he continued.

"Watch the moon when it moves from east to west, right to left. There, in the middle of the direction is the north. It will bring you to Ohio, to your freedom!"

While listening to his father the little boy also peered into the sky and tried to figure out the direction.

"There, dad?", he asked inquisitively, pointing in the direction described by his father.

"Yes, that is the door to your freedom. Never forget that, son!" replied his father in a steady voice.

Since that day, his father's words remained firmly etched in his memory. He watched the moon until the day his father passed away when

Moon Watcher was a young man. His father was the closest person and his only living relative. He never saw his mother because she died in childbirth.

Gently, he opened his eyes, and with shaky knees, he moved toward the chair, taking deep breaths with every step.

As he moved forward he remembered his last beating after his failed attempt to run away from the plantation.

"Now, Moon Watcher! You'll get the lesson of your life. You'll never run away again!" his master exclaimed with a look of hatred in his eyes. Turning to his worker, he nodded.

By now, Moon Watcher already knew what to expect. He took a deep breath and immediately pain tore through his already battered body. The look of anxiety spread across his face as he prepared to take the next blow.

"Huuuu! Huuuu! Huuuu! Lord, please have mercy on me!" was uttered after every blow.

It would seem like hours before the beating would cease, but the weeks, months and years of pain and agony from his injuries would seem even worse than a single beating alone.

Moon Watcher prepared for the next blow to come, but the pain that would ravage through his body this time would be worse than he could ever imagine. A white man, one of his master's workers, stood behind Moon Watcher while he was still fettered and raised an iron hammer high in the air. With much strength, the hammer descended onto Moon Watchers legs. A horrifying and painful cry was heard as if it were the releasing of Moon Watcher's soul. His screaming could be heard for miles.

He imagined watching himself as he was being beaten by his master after being caught attempting to run away from the plantation. He saw his

arms and legs tied with heavy iron chains as he tried to free himself. At the end of his beating, there would be blood all over his injured back.

At the age of six he was put to work as a slave on the plantation. He worked hard from dawn till dusk and Jived in an environment where slave men, women and children were horrifically treated and given meagre wages. Sometimes they would only receive bread, black beans, water and nothing else. Each night he fell asleep due to mere exhaustion.

For years, he had to endure the violations of the integrity of black people such as mutilation, physical and mental torture, undue psychological pressures, and subhuman living conditions. He had now come to a point in his life where he was literally tired of being a slave.

He would be crippled for the rest of his life. A man who was once strong and a prime of life at the age of fifty-five. He had not only lost adequate physical means of mobility, but his mind was shattered, he had become mentally disabled. His life was pure torture. He suffered from recurring panic attacks, day after day and night after night if any thought brought to his mind the day he became a cripple. His soul was completely desecrated. There was no human dignity left, and no way out for him from being a slave except one.

He stopped before the chair and slowly managed to climb up. He then shoved his head into the hole, pulling the rope until it was taut. Lowering his voice he began to pray.

"Lord, forgive me! Bring me to my family, to a better place where my soul will be in peace!"

In the last moments of his life, an expression of contentment flashed across his face and with determination, he sprang from the chair. At first

his body started to shake fiercely and his feet began to tremble. Eventually, silence filled the room.

Finally, his soul was released from all torture, and he could rest in peace as he always wanted to.

SLAVERY AND MENTAL HEALTH

Slavery in the Unites States of America begun in the 17th century when the first Africans were shipped to Virginia to work as indentured servants on the plantation. As time passed, wealthy whites from the north ventured into the trade of selling slaves to land owners in the south which resulted in shipment of more blacks to the western world. Unlike other slaves, the indentured servants exercised some degree of freedom since their services were based upon a voluntary agreement.

Slaves offered a great deal of inexpensive labor on tobacco, rice, and indigo plantations (Williams 2013). Eventually at least one third of the southern population was comprised of slaves. Through laws called 'slave codes', the slaves were denied the opportunity to learn how to read and write and, as a result, became heavily dependent on their owners. Slave owners controlled their slaves and slaves were subjected to brutality if any of them failed to follow orders.

In 1868, the 14th Amendment granted black Americans citizenship and some civil rights. Among those rights was the right to vote. In the following years, the physical walls of slavery deteriorated, and it was condemned in most states, but most blacks remained in poverty. Most of them became sharecroppers; renting land by sharing their crops with landowners to make a living for their families. Freed slaves were subject to poor living conditions that, in turn, affected their health. Today, black Americans still live in poverty and experience an extreme disparity of resources.

Despite the efforts to ensure equal distribution of resources, African Americans continue to lack quality educational, medical, and financial

resources. Although blacks have greatly contributed to the economic growth of America, they are constantly faced with racial discrimination. Though, with time, blacks have migrated to other parts of the country, a vast majority of the African American population still reside in the southern part of the country where slavery was largely practiced. This region is characterized by high crime rates, unemployment, few resources, and homelessness.

In states with a large population of black Americans, violence and crime rates are high and there is a high occurrence of single parent homes. Raising a child in such an environment increase the possibilities of having a traumatic experience, affects their way of thinking, and may hinder effective brain development. Therefore, mental health is highly influenced by one's upbringing. Such trauma faced by children in these environments contributes to the high rates of mental illnesses within the black community.

In 1969, members of the American Psychiatric Association (APA) brought up the issue of racial discrimination in mental clinics where the black Americans did not receive equal medical attention as whites (APA, 2013). Among them were the black psychiatrists Drs. J. A. Cannon, James P. Comer, Chester M. Pierce, James Ralph and Charles Wilkerson. They protested by demanding the inclusion of black psychiatrists in influential positions of the APA so that people of color could be represented well, and to ensure that they received adequate medical care. A facet of the response to their protest included the construction of additional medical facilities in the rural areas, with the hiring and training of black medical professionals. White psychiatrists were encouraged to equally attend to the black patients as they would white patients and membership was denied to those who refused. One of the direct results was that the number of black

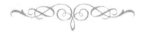

patients increased; however, barriers remained for blacks to seek proper mental health treatment.

Unlike most in the black community, many white Americans have access to insurance, belong to the middle class, and have access to quality medical facilities; whereas most blacks live below the poverty line and lack these amenities. Additionally, stigma amongst black Americans makes it difficult for them to seek medical assistance after they have developed a mental illness. Some may be rendered helpless or develop unrealistic ideologies as to whether or not they are able to improve. Others seek alternate methods of dealing with their mental issues. Furthermore, most black Americans do not acknowledge their mental problems which affect their ability to cope (Ward et al, 2013). Because of the perception that white therapists lack the personal experiences that are necessary when dealing with mental illnesses among the blacks, some blacks avoid seeking the help that is needed.

Slavery has played a very important role in the development of mental health issues. Although the topic of slavery remains taboo in modem day America, for African Americans the topic evokes emotions of embarrassment and anger, and in most cases, affects their relations with whites. On the other hand, some white Americans may feel guilt. Extensive research and discussion about the enslavement of African Americans would be the first step to healing. Next, we must identify the factors that heavily contribute to the disparities between white and black Americans, and then recommend the best measures to be implemented to overcome these challenges.

DRAPETOMANIA: SLAVE SICKNESS

In 1849, Samuel Adolphus Cartwright, a physician, was assigned the task by the Louisiana Medical Convention of observing the unique behavior of African-Americans. He titled his research 'Disease and Physical Peculiarities of the Negro Race'. In his research, Cartwright developed the name Drapetomania as the mental disease that caused slaves to run away from their masters. Cartwright criticized all white slave owners of their attempts to treat blacks as equals, or for denying their necessities because he believed that this was the cause of this mental illness. Cartwright's research presented blacks as a people never in need of freedom, instead, they were pictured as victims of this mental disorder if they desired freedom.

To support his theories, Cartwright argued that black people had smaller brains and sensitive skin compared to their white counterparts. He correlated these differences with the idea that blacks were not descendants of Adam and Eve which seemingly justified that the right place for the slave was to remain a slave. Cartwright described slaves as submissive knee benders who should not be treated as human beings and further argued that any attempt for the white man to treat a slave as his equal was an abuse of the power given to him by God. Any attempt to live a life contrary to this idea was considered a sign of mental illness.

Cartwright's research did not only criticize slave owners who failed to provide for the basic necessities of their slaves, and failed in protecting them from abuse, but it suggested a treatment for this illness. He theorized that the illness was curable if only the white man would exercise his full

powers over the black slaves and deny them an opportunity to feel human. He explained that blacks who became dissatisfied with their master's failure to provide for their basic needs were more likely to run away, therefore, slave owners were encouraged to determine if the slaves reason for being dissatisfied was genuine and reasonable. If the reason found was genuine and reasonable in the eyes of the owner, then they were encouraged to look for ways to solve it. However, Cartwright suggested that if the reason was not genuine then the 'devil should be whipped out' of the slave. This was also seen as a preventative measure for other slaves who thought to run away or behave disorderly.

These ideas presented by Cartwright were widely criticized by northern whites, whereas the southern whites embraced this idea. Rather than these suggestions being used only as a treatment, they were widely used to prevent slaves from running away. Most slaves were subjected to torture to ensure that they remained submissive. This would serve as an example to the other slaves who may have desired their freedom.

Cartwright's medical advice to white slave owners was to cut the toes off the slaves and severely whip them to return them to a submissive state. This would also be a way to ensure that slaves would remain on the plantation because they would lose their ability to walk effectively. The pain caused by such punishment birthed fear in the hearts of the slaves which served to continually remind them of their inferiority to their white slave masters and any idea of equality to white was extinguished.

Cartwright was an advocate for slavery and justified the institution of Slavery by arguing that blacks benefited from it, and were crazy if they tried to escape. White oppressors believed that they were doing their slaves a great favor by providing food, clothing, and shelter. However, there was no

mistaking who was really being benefitted from the institution of Slavery. White slave owners grew wealthier while blacks suffered in poverty, were overworked, declined in health, and were taken away from their families and sold to other oppressors against their will. He further challenged those who sought to abolish slavery by attributing their influences to misguided ideas.

Many southern American natives considered black people, especially those born in Africa, very inferior and incapable of performing certain duties. To prove this theory, they looked for scientific proof which was mainly based on their observation of blacks such as their color, culture, and behaviors. Most of the whites considered blacks lazy and believed that their goal was to drain their financial resources while in reality, blacks were the greatest contributors to their financial success. In the northern region, slavery was not as popular, but they shipped Africans to America and sold them to southern plantation owners as a source of income. Therefore, both regions benefited financially from the institution of slavery in the western world.

These theories about African Americans that were presented by Cartwright have been criticized as an observation for the political class. Some have described it as psychopathology that was influenced by racism, culture, politics, and not science. His main aim was to stop activists from demanding for the equal rights of blacks and impede congress' actions in passing the amendments that granted African Americans equal right as whites. In his letter, featured in the DeBow's Review, titled 'How to Save the Republic, and Position of the South in the Union', Cartwright politically criticizes African countries and northern abolitionists. With the Southern Union falling apart due to the increased demands to end slavery,

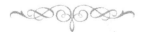

Cartwright's report was a means of saving it and helping others who shared his beliefs. What he attributed to Drapetomania, other physicians describe as a result of poverty and exposure to violence.

There were some who believed that the conclusions of Cartwright's research was valid and continued his research to prove the inferiority of the African American people. Later, in the 1960s, Vernom Mark, William Sweet, and Frank Ervin suggested that 'brain dysfunction' was the reason blacks protested in urban areas and caused violence. In order to reduce this violence, they introduced the idea of 'psychosurgery' (William, 2013). Other psychiatrists such as Drs. Alvin Poussaint and Peter Breggin, who supported black freedom, went to the streets to protest against this suggestion. Many blacks rejected the white man's god and established unique beliefs that connected with their social and historical experiences. This gave them hope and strength to keep pressing forward. During the period of the Underground Railroad, many blacks joined abolitionists in the south in the fight for the freedom of blacks and assisting them in finding freedom.

MENTAL HEALTH CARE AND AFRICAN AMERICAN SLAVE MEN

Mental health care among African American men has been a topic of discussion for a number of years. One of the factors that contribute to this ongoing discussion is the diverse experiences that they have that make them more vulnerable to developing psychological disorders. There are many factors that contribute to poor mental health for men of color. Some factors include environment, economic and social challenges, and racial discrimination (Erlanger, 2017). We will explore these contributors and possible solutions to these conditions.

Causes of Mental Illness

First, we will discuss the effect of environment and its social and economic challenges on mental health. When we compare predominantly black communities with communities with a predominantly white population, black communities present challenges for men of color to raise adequate finances to provide the daily necessities of their families. The communities are flooded with violence, poverty, neglect, and abuse, which increases mental stress. This also increases to possibility of traumatic situations occurring in the home. Many young men in these environments experience anxiety and are at a higher risk of developing a mental illness.

Second, discrimination has also become a culprit in the decline of mental health among black men. Much discrimination comes from Jaw enforcement, working environment, and sometimes recreational facilities. With the increase in experiences of discrimination, victims develop low

self-esteem and guilt. The latter makes it difficult to engage with others resulting in a feeling of loneliness. Feeling segregated from the general public creates much stress to the victim and discourages them from visiting clinical facilities in search of proper therapeutic services.

A third contributor to poor mental health is racial injustice. History reveals occurrences of racial injustices from both members of the public, and law enforcement, of which African American males are the greatest victims. When we consider racial injustice experienced from law enforcement, it is safe to assume that when an individual does not feel safe with the institution that is meant to protect them, it creates an insecurity which, in tum, contributes to some level of stress. When stress gradually increases from different sources, it may lead to various mental illnesses which, in turn, means poor overall mental health in the society. Black American males are often perceived as dangerous and are sometimes killed when being confronted by law enforcement (Geller, 2014). The Journal of Public Health further confirms that those who survive racial injustice from encounters with law enforcement are at higher risk for post• traumatic stress disorder.

Other significant contributors to poor health among the African American male includes genetics, and family history.

Stigma

Stigma refers to a label of disgrace that is associated with a particular individual or group within the society, and there exists a stigma towards black American males. Black males are not just considered to be more violent, but they are seen as contributors to their mental condition and are not given adequate support in order to assist them in seeking proper

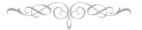

mental health care. The number of easily accessible mental health care facilities to African American residents are fewer than those accessible to white Americans, despite the fact that the Blacks are more likely develop a mental illness.

Additionally, despite the increase in the number of mental health care facilities, there are fewer African American therapists. This results in fewer black men seeking mental health care because there is believed to be a lack of familiarity. Some perceive black therapists as those who understand the plight of other African Americans. Very little encouragement is given to black men to ensure mental health diagnosis is conducted and this facilitates ignorance toward mental health in African American males.

Mistreatment and Misdiagnosis

Much evidence exists concerning misdiagnosis or mistreatment of African American patients by health care professionals. Studies indicate that black people are misdiagnosed with severe psychological disorders/ conditions despite comparative behaviors shown among whites that receive a less severe diagnosis. Such misfortunes discourage black men from taking advantage of mental health care facilities as there may be a misinterpretation of their condition. Mistreating of clients by service providers also discourages future enquiries from those who may need the attention of a mental health professional.

Lack of Culturally Informed Care

African American males are generally encouraged to be self-reliant, and are often the weight bearers of their struggles. As a result of this, many

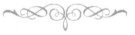

of them do not seek the necessary help needed to address their mental conditions. Furthermore, black men who develop low self-esteem do not engage freely with others, and lack adequate knowledge of the state of their mental health. Inadequate awareness in addition to cultural misinformation plays a vital role in few black men seeking mental health care.

Ways to Enhance Mental Health Care

Introduce Platforms to Disclose Information

Public awareness is a critical tool in improving public health. Currently, the advancement of technology can be used to enhance and transfer information to the public. Social media can be used to communicate the necessary information about various mental health issues, their signs, prevention and treatment, and the location of appropriate facilities to aid in treatment. Additionally, educational programs can be conducted to target African American men to provide them with adequate information on mental health.

Encourage More Black Men in Research

As mentioned above, black men prefer to be treated by black therapists. Improving the health of the public, which includes that of African Americans, requires for more black men to be encouraged to become involved in the research industry. It solves not only the health issue but also encourages confidence among the African American in seeking mental health care. It improves their level of openness and provides unobstructed access to the culturally complex health issues.

Black men should further be encouraged to change their perception of mental health care. This can be achieved by creating massive public awareness and taking steps to prevent current victimization and stigmatization. Discouraging police brutality and providing help for those struggling with feelings of guilt and low self-esteem offers an opportunity for black men, who are mostly impacted, to be able to express their mental health concerns without fear and stigmatization. When the perusal of mental

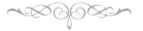

health assistance is no longer equated with weakness and vulnerability, black men will begin to embrace the opportunities provided for mental health care. Moreover, it would benefit black men to avoid the idea that only black therapists are competent to provide adequate treatment because both blacks and white are equally competent.

Mental health medical professionals should undergo regular training to educate them on the importance of accurate diagnosis and proper treatment of black male clients. Such a step improves the confidence of black males who seek attention in mental health facilities. Close monitoring should be done to ensure that black male clients are not mistreated for this not only discourages them from pursuing medical treatment, but also deprives them of their human right to fair treatment and good health. In essence, in order to improve the mental health of black men, one must seek ways of eradicating the various obstacles involved. Good governance in public health facilities, properly qualified professionals to provide health services, and excellent working relationship can serve the purpose adequately.

MENTAL HEALTH AND AFRICAN AMERICAN SLAVE WOMEN

Many women, regardless of race, have experiences that increase their risks for developing a mental illness and other related disorders. Therefore, effective and early intervention is essential in order to ensure the condition does not become incapable of being managed. Just as African American males, black women face similar challenges in accessing effective, adequate, and affordable mental health care. Amidst the challenges they may face, and the character of selfless sacrifice for the wellbeing of their children shown by most mothers, black women appear as figures of strength to their families and communities. This usually comes at an expensive cost.

Causes of Mental Illness

There are no exclusive causes of mental illness for the African American women. However, the most common type of mental illness affecting black women is depression. Depression can be cause by the loss of a loved one, environmental, economic, or social issues.

Another factor that contributes to mental illness is genetics. A woman who has a family history of mental illness has an increased possibility of becoming a victim of a similar mental condition in her lifetime. Though heredity may play a part to the repeated occurrence, it is not an apparent cause. Social• economic factors may cause mental illness. This includes the current surrounding they are exposed to because it may cause stress, if the surrounding is more violent or there are poor living conditions. The severity of the surroundings also increases the likelihood that these

black women can be exposed to traumatic situations. Trauma alone causes mental instability and contributed to stress which may lead into a state of depression.

Effect of Age Difference on African American Women

Despite age being a minor factor considered in mental health, within black women, age affects how they perceive psychological health. Younger black women do not rely so heavily on religious beliefs in comparison to older black women. Additionally, exposure to technology provides access to much information which shifts the beliefs of the young away from customs and traditions. Whereas older black women endorse treatment seeking while mid-age and young women endorse avoidance coping.

Barriers to Mental Illness Treatment

Despite the fact that black women are often faced with the burden of psychological illness, most do not take advantage of psychiatric services (Mathew & Hughes, 2001). This is attributed to the fact that there are various beliefs associated with mental illness. In the 1990s, a study showed that African American women viewed those with depression as weak and as a dangerous. Moreover, it was believed that they had a small mind, lack of self-love as well as troubled spirits. Later on, Thompson-Sanders found that African Americans connected mental illness with embarrassment and shame which influences those with any form of mental illness to be hid from the public. Also, some black woman believed that they were not vulnerable to depression. These wide range of beliefs discourage black women from seeking much needed mental health care. Such ideas

are influenced by popular beliefs of what it means to be a 'strong black women', which have persisted over the last few decades.

Distrust of Medical Interventions

A few years ago, the black community was used to test new medication. This created much discomfort in black communities and the negative attitude generated has extended to current generations where black women fear they may be used as an experiment in testing new medication and practices. Therefore, most African American women fear the discrimination that exists in the health sectors. Distrust also occurs when black woman experience a cultural disconnect between them and their health providers. It is feared that this may affect the way in which therapists offer their services (Whaley, 2001). Such barrier in culture reduces the client's tendency to stay and seek treatment. Needless to mention, through history there is distrust of the US health system as a result of victimization and traumatic experiences of black women.

Lack of Information

Some African American women are not fully aware of what mental health care entails. Due to the popular correlation of psychological difficulties and shame, from the stigmatization point of view, many shy away from this topic. Being exposed to little information presents numerous problems which not only becomes a barrier, but also denies them a chance to benefit from services. They lack information to know when and where to find needed mental health care services, and find trouble in identifying signs and symptoms of the psychological illness. This makes it quite easy

to underestimate the potential impact avoiding intervention will have on the victim of mental illness.

Faith, Spirituality, and Community

Family and spiritual beliefs are the main foundations of support and strength for the African American woman and within society at large. When faced with emotional and other stressful conditions, black women rely on religious based relationships rather than medical treatment. Indeed, sometimes these connections are beneficial, but it should not be the only option. There exists a number of instances where the psychological condition has been left unrecognized by faith based relations. Therefore, beliefs in the community and faith can also become a barrier to seeking mental health care.

Socio-Economic Factors

Some black women, due to their level of poverty, may decide not to seek medical attention in order to save for other basic needs. A survey by US Census Bureau (2012) suggests that less African American women have health insurance coverage despite poverty and high vulnerability to mental illness. Therefore, socio-economics creates difficulty in accessing quality mental health care even after they receive a diagnosis.

Biases and Inequality of Care

Some mental health practitioners are biased in providing health checkups to African American women. This encourages a decline in the number of black women seeking medical coverage or services. It also

proliferates mistrust unless given good providers who will give better and reliable information and treatment.

Coping Method

Employing different tactics will help to assist black women with managing mental illnesses. One of these tactics is to adopt a women's support system that develops friendly relationships. These support groups will seek to provide a safe environment for women to openly discuss issues that may seem shameful or embarrassing. Sharing life experiences provides opportunity to exchange ideas of coping with mental disorders among friends (Oakley, 2005). It provides an alternative voice of reason and fosters compassion to take on and achieve life goals more readily.

Creating mental illness awareness programs for women by health professionals is another better alternative. Awareness comes in handy to solve many spheres of the issues associated with mental health care. It provides answers to highly debated questions concerning mental health care such as the level of discrimination that African American women are subjected to. Moreover, it provides a platform for responding to these queries. When mental health experts of different races provide guidance in an open and friendly arena, it improves the confidence of black women in the health system as well as improves patient-therapist relationships.

Use of technology is also a better way of addressing the mental health problem. Black Public Media is a useful platform in targeting and perhaps eliminating the issue of stigmatization. Eradicating stigma within the community pushes it in a direction to heal and address problems head-on without fear of not receiving adequate assistance. It results in a culture shift which discourages loneliness among black women, and fostering an

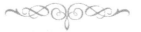

environment filled with friends who empower one another. This will make the difference when seeking to improve the state of mental health care within the African American community.

In conclusion, mental health care is vital for both men and women. There are various factors within the African American community that make them more vulnerable to mental illnesses than whites. Numerous barriers are developed which significantly affect the access to mental health care for African Americans as discussed above. For black women, the firm belief and spiritual alignment may make it difficult for them to access mental health care. Many in the African American community suffer from low self-esteem, fear of discrimination, and have distrust toward therapists which causes them to dislike seeking mental health care facilities. With time, technology has come to aid in creating awareness and closing the cultural gap which makes it difficult to access medical care. It is crucial that African Americans seek mental health assistance for it is of great benefit.

PSYCHOPATHOLOGY IN THE AFRICAN AMERICAN COMMUNITY

Without sound psychological health one cannot be considered a healthy individual. Many people experience ups and downs due to the many events they experience in their lives. Mental health goes beyond these emotional reactions to specific situations. They include medical conditions that affect our feelings and the way we think. These changes can alter one's life in ways that places pressure on the victim's relationships with others, thus causing them to malfunction.

Although anyone can experience these changes, African-Americans sometimes suffer more severely from mental illness due to barriers and other unmet needs. They are 200% more likely to experience psychological illhealth than the general population. About 2.3 million Americans have bipolar disorder, also referred to as the manic-depressive illness. The African-American community is even less likely to receive a diagnosis and hence treatment for this disease although it is common among them (Schnittker, Freese & Powell, 2013). This research study aiming to discover risk factors for developing mental disorder, its prevalence among the African-American community, signs and symptoms, and behavioral aspects brought about by this mental condition.

Behaviors Associated with Mental Disorders

Several aspects and practices are believed to be associated with psychiatric disorders both in adults, children, and adolescents. These include the following:

Anxiety and Substance Abuse

Diagnostic and prospective studies have been conducted on adults, children, and adolescents. These studies provided casual associations between anxiety and substance abuse. Violation of these substances was found to increase vulnerability to anxiety by exerting a physiological effect on the brain of the user. Stress also may reduce or delay the problem of substance abuse by reminding the user of its impact and consequences of using them. Moreover, it may cause one to develop or sustain a substance use disorder as a way of managing anxiety.

Several studies conducted on this group have found that Self-Medications Thesis is highly associated with this problem. Persons with anxiety use alcohol and other narcotic drugs to suppress their symptoms of anxiety. It was primarily found to be the case in girls compared to boys by Costello et al. Some studies also found that substance abuse promoted the development of anxiety in these age groups. Later, those with fear started smoking. Each type of stress was associated with unique behavioral outcomes for each person within those categories.

Depression and Substance Abuse

Adults, children, and adolescents in the African-American community have abused substances as a way of self-medication to manage symptoms of depression, or to change their behavior under various circumstances. Substance abuse may lead to increase in vulnerability to depression, and use of marijuana was associated with depression.

Sign and Symptom of Mental Illness Observed

Studies revealed that within African American communities, abnormal activity level was common among patients with a behavioral disorder. Some were distracted by the objects and people around them. These activities include:

Hyperactivity

It was observed that those with this condition rushed from doing one task to another without fully completing tasks. When handling the second task they realized they did not complete the previous task and, without relaxing, they rush to complete the first task. In the end, nothing is done properly. They lacked concentration, organization, and time management in performing each task and, therefore, were unable to accomplish the necessary tasks. Without proper intervention, their condition worsens, and they may become unable to properly function in the broader society.

Hypoactivity

Most of the African-American communities observed with mental illness appeared reluctant, reserved, and were involved in very little activity. When their condition became severe, they remained idle for hours, accomplishing little even the simplest of household or personal hygiene chores. Most had slow and limited speech, thoughts, they exhibit immobility, and appear terrified most of the time.

Akathisia

It is a case that was evident in most of the subjects, for instance mostly those in late adolescence showed a state of motor restlessness. This group demonstrated an inability to be still or sited. Their muscles became restless and difficult to coordinate for various activities. They developed behavior of retracting their steps, march in place and sit, stand and then sit again. They could perform the same action repeatedly.

Mannerism

The groups affected with this condition showed some old behaviors, they could make some mistake intentionally or accidentally. Though this is expected in many teenagers, theirs was met with reluctance and rudeness, so to say. They became angry and mute when asked about the behaviors. When they recovered, some could not explain their actions and only had a vague memory of what occurred.

Gait Problems

In each case that was observed, musculoskeletal disease, impairment of neurologic tissues and psychiatric disorder were observed. Depressive illness affected gait by slowing it, others included intoxication by sedative drugs, hypothyroidism, and frontal, temporal dementia. Those who chronically abused stimulant drugs exhibited a jerky bird-like gait.

The Prevalence of the Disorder Based on the Study

According to a survey conducted by Bonnie Duran et al. on substance use, mood, anxiety and somatoform disorder prevalence, 89% of the total

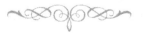

population depended on marijuana or had abused this drug in their lifetime. Cocaine is the second most widely reported drug of choice. 65% had an alcohol problem in their life (Swartz et al, 2015). Marijuana accounted for 80% of drug abuse or dependence. Prevalence of any mood disorder was 44%, with 86% of the women with mood disorder suffering from major depression. Almost all the women had bipolar I disorder.

The most common mental disorder was anxiety. 62.8% of the African-Americans in the study met criteria for any lifetime anxiety disorder diagnosis. The most common anxiety disorders were phobias, and post-traumatic stress, 59% of the study participants had the disease according to Bonnie Duran et al. in their study. Of the particular neuroses, the animal type was most common, followed by natural environment, then blood injection injury. The most common somatoform disorder was conversion disorder with 2.5% for both lifetime and past-year (Alegria et al., 2012). Among those who reported any lifetime diagnosis of depression, 8.2% had lifetime anxiety disorder, and 54% had experienced depression.

Risk factors Associated with Mental Disorders

Those with lower education levels tend to develop these mental disorders due to more moderate self-esteem they applied on themselves. They felt discriminated and abandoned in the society hence, in the long run, establish negative feeling about life and everything in their surroundings.

Studies revealed that African Americans that experienced homelessness are at a higher risk of developing a mental health condition, of which they make up around 40o/o of the homeless population. Moreover, exposure to violence increased the risk of developing a mental health problem. Such problems include depression, anxiety, and post-traumatic stress disorder.

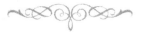

In this case, the African American children were at higher risk than white children.

Conclusion

The higher prevalence of the psychiatric disorders as noted in the present study may be attributed to factors such as: drug abuse (use of cocaine and marijuana), substance abuse, environmental and demographic factors, which influence mental and physical behaviors. The disorders are seen mostly affecting toddlers, children, and teenagers. Based on the study males are changed more compared to women by these diseases. They always want to prove themselves to the opposite sex, and in the process, they get carried away by the behavior, leading to addiction hence as explained, the relationship between substance abuse and disorders.

DEPRESSION, NEUROSIS, AND PERSONALITY DISORDERS IN THE AFRICAN AMERICAN COMMUNITY

Depression

Depression is a condition that results when an individual undergoes intense levels of stress that may cause the affected individual to lose the sense of life. High levels of depression may influence the individual to attempt suicide. Depression is a major disabling disorder affecting African American communities. So many beliefs among African Americans discourages them from seeking necessary mental health care. According to USA Department of Health and Human Services Offices of Minority Services, African Americans have a high likelihood of about 20% of having severe depression than other races in the American population (Mata et al., 2015). A number of reasons increase the chances of avoiding seeking medical attention regardless of age. Below are some factors that increase chances of developing severe cases of depression for African Americans.

Stigma

Different myths of shame and embarrassment exist among BlackAmericans. These bring much confusion as well as unnecessary pain as victims of depression have no place to ease the burden of such a condition. So many blacks rely on the family, faith and community in matters of emotional imbalance hence avoid mental facilities (Mata et al., 2015). They believe that one should take their problems to Jesus

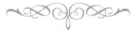

only, rather than seeking the professional assistance that has been made available. This is a dire misconception and a cultural misunderstanding that can lead to severe problems. There is fear of exposing their problems to someone else and fear that people may look down on them upon discovery of their condition. This also acts as a barrier towards treating their mental conditions.

Lack of Knowledge

Despite the fact that some platforms foster awareness and encourage competence in the area of mental health for the larger community, many individuals within the black community lack knowledge of its existence. This lack of knowledge about mental health issues places them at a disadvantage and renders them victims of these severe conditions. Little information leads to trouble in identifying signs and symptoms of the depression hence undervaluing the potential effects of not looking for support. Many African Americans usually don't know what mental health care entails and its overall benefits.

Social Economic Factors

Some environmental conditions increase chances of being in depression as well as avoidance of seeking medical attention. According to a study conducted in 2012, around 40% of homeless populations was African American (Mata et al., 2015). They also live in a place where violence is rampant which increases chances of depression. Furthermore, they live in high poverty conditions as compared to their white counterparts. Such living conditions discourage mental health assistance as they prefer catering for basic needs over seeking medical assistance. Most African

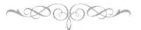

Americas have no medical coverage to help them access treatment for depression (Mata et al., 2015).

Mistrust Among Clinicians

Some studies show that therapists tend to be discriminative against Blacks. African Americans feel uneasy to visit them despite having signs of depression. Misdiagnosis added to mistrust increases levels of depression as seeking psychological treatment becomes impossible (McWilliams, 2011). Lack or fewer numbers of Black therapists compound the problem of increased depression. Blacks feel they do not have people whom they share same social dynamics and can understand them well.

Cultural

Many African Americans promote an image that perceives them as healthy. The idea of a "strong black woman" and the "masculine black man" who should not show their feelings to the society makes it difficult to treat African Americans. They overlook the need for mental health care as they feel ready enough to tackle life's hurdles whatever the circumstance. There is an increased belief of being invincible to depression.

Neurosis

It is a mental disorder that involves chronic distress with no hallucinations and delusions. Examples of neuroses are impulse control disorder, obsessive-compulsive disorder, and anxiety disorder. Many African Americans, just like the general population, suffers from neuroses disorder. There are no unique causes of neurosis in blacks, however, there

are situations which make neurosis disorder more severe in African Americas (Russon, 2003). Below is a discussion of these conditions.

Some African American community members content themselves with wrong or insufficient answers to life questions. According to Jung's theory of neurosis, individuals having existential issues are likely to suffer from neurosis (Russon, 2003). Black Americans thinking of having answers to their psychological condition, and failing to seek mental assistance, increase their likelihood of amplified neurosis. Also, the lack of solutions in the surrounding environment where black Americans live increases pressure in their life which causes an alteration in the psyche, emotional state of an individual.

Neurosis may occur from the need of an ego defense mechanism. It involves the development and maintaining of a sense of self-respect and existence. African Americas feels the need to protect themselves from those who they think to look down on them. Needless to mention, neurosis in Blacks is a by-product of racism. It is in this sense that African Americans feel disappointed and stressed when a police officer stops them. The idea that the police officer stopped an individual because they are black is a neurotic condition as there are many reasons for this and is often necessary in their work. In psychoanalytical theory, the need of developing ego defense mechanism can lead a person to experience unconscious conflict and emotional distress which is a part of neurosis.

An environment where one lives and those they live with play a vital role in the development of unstable mental conditions. In this case, African Americans build an idealized image from experiences, particular needs, as well as earlier fantasies. Such cause of increased neurosis in Blacks is

evident in Homey's theory of neurosis where she offers an array of ways to fight neurosis.

Personality Disorder

A personality disorder is a mental illness identified by having unhealthy and a rigid behavior, thinking, and functioning (Connolly, 2008). Examples of personality disorders affecting African Americans are antisocial, schizoid, schizotypal, paranoia, histrionic and borderline personality disorder.

An individual with a personality disorder experiences troubles in relating (interpersonal function), impulse control and perceiving the different situations and people. The condition is associated with distress and disability. Those suffering from the disorder have a personal coping problem which leads to grief, depression or extreme anxiety and there are factors that place African Americans at risk.

Abusive Environment

Raising a child in a chaotic environment increases the chance of developing a personality disorder (Connolly, 2008). Some families are unstable and chaotic leaving all members to endure harsh conditions in life. Such environments increase emotional instability and stress among members exposed to violence. Such life situations make victims vulnerable to personality disorders as they cannot control the patterns of their living.

Related Illnesses

Exposure to mental illnesses makes people vulnerable to developing a personality disorder. African American family situations, like living an isolated life, present a viable ground for personality disorder. By any chance, if a person has depression, they may develop personality disorder as they try to cope. Studies show that Blacks are susceptible to other mental illness and heredity is a factor that increases this possibility.

Parenting Issues

Evidence shows that personality disorder starts from the parent'spersonality disorder then pass on to children. Many African Americans find it difficult to achieve higher education, securing right relationships, as well as obtaining steady jobs in the society. Their children can begin to develop personality disorder during such difficult states experienced by their parents. Furthermore, poor parenting among some African American families shows elevated levels of vulnerability to personality disorders. When a maternal relationship is not adequately fostered within the African American community, later in life, it leads to the development of a personality disorder.

Just like many other mental illnesses, African Americans finds it difficult to pursue personality disorder health care. The fear of victimization acts as a barrier, and the lack of black therapists who understand the plight of living in the political and social system discourages African Americans from seeking mental health care when needed. Lack of reliable information about the disease and importance of trying mental health care is devastating.

A therapist can employ several methods to increase African American enquires of personality disorder treatments. Family therapy becomes vital as it controls the likelihood of transmitting the same problems from parent to child. There should be self-help groups which will foster a conducive environment to discuss personality disorders treatment programs and provide prerequisite information.

Lastly, mindfulness among the therapist has become an excellent clinical tool to treat personality disorder among African Americans as it increases their confidence in the mental health care system.

POVERTY AND MENTAL HEALTH DISORDERS

Mental health disorder has a direct relationship with poverty. The severity of mental illness is more evident in those perceived as inferior as compared to those who are not. An overwhelming number of individuals living with mental illness get little attention in psychiatric facilities, due to lack of finances to cater to their needs. However, there is no clear explanation on which precedes the other, is it poverty or mental illness. Nevertheless, poverty, through many research studies, is a risk factor to mental illness. For one to promote mental health care, they should first address the question of poverty in the society as the two issues are intertwined.

According to the general public, poverty can be defined as a lack of sufficient income or wealth to provide the necessities of life like health care, education, and shelter. Poverty is estimated by how far any individual falls below the poverty line. Understanding this definition lays the foundation upon which one discusses the direct relationship between poverty and mental disorder. So many mental diseases are associated with poverty, however, schizophrenia has less likelihood of association with poverty.

How Poverty Increases Mental Health Disorder Vulnerability

Poverty creates barriers to proper mental health care. Specific elements associated with poverty include:

Income

A sustainable income from whichever source improves people's living standards. At the point where individuals lack a source of income, it translates into the origin of poverty. Income generating projects are linked with a steady and permanent employment. Currently, some citizens depend on the part-time job, thus living on a pay check to pay check kind of life. Furthermore, work raises one's self• esteem hence attaching a social meaning as well as providing the fundamental needs of their families.

Therefore, it translates that when an individual doesn't have an employment position nor has any income generating project, they lack means to cater for mental health care. Depression, one of the significant psychological disorders is linked to low self-esteem (Mc Williams, 2011). Naturally, when someone is depressed and does not have that courage to share their condition, they end up in the severe level of the disorder. Finances are a vital ingredient to better mental health care, therefore, little or no income results in not seeking quality mental health care or indigent health care, if one manages to pursue it.

Mental Illness Affecting Employment and Income

When one is diagnosed with mental illness, it affects their capabilities in conducting their duties effectively and efficiently. In workstations, some levels of stigmatization occur. Those who have mental illnesses are assumed as a burden in the workplace and usually find themselves in poverty when asked or driven to quit or lose a work contract. They end up living exclusively on the disability allowance. As a result of mental health issues in the work environment, and the stigmatization that follows,

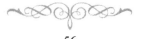

those who are incapable of surviving with the workplace pressures, are inevitably lead into unemployment.

Education

Poor people have an average lesser level of education than those considered wealthy. Education plays a significant role in creating awareness about mental health diseases, their signs and symptoms, as well as treatment. Among the main reasons behind lack of seeking medical and psychological assistance is lack of knowledge. It is therefore right to conclude that those who do not have higher education may become vulnerable to mental illness. They do not recognize the need to pursue psychological treatment and the benefits associated with it. Lack of knowledge influences one to avoid treatment and provides minimal opportunities to seek mental checkup and therapy which, in turn, increases levels of mental illness.

Furthermore, high education increases the chances of securing better employment. As stated above, lack of jobs leads to low income, hence increase the risk of poverty. Persons whose level of education is low or else outdated are subjected to low-income employment. It perpetuates the poverty life cycle in their families, hence acting as a barrier toward access to resources needed to support their well• being and mental and medical health care.

Mental Illness Effects on Education

Sometimes mental illness strikes at the age of adolescence or early adulthood. At that time, an individual is undertaking formal education. It leads to interruptions in their education, thus lowering future chances of acquiring a good job. Also, mental disorders may cause abandonment of

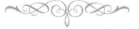

school, making it difficult to obtain sufficient training and preparation to function in the society in the future. It adds to the level of poverty in the community in the long run.

Housing

Proper, safe and affordable housing is pivotal in a stable life and the perusal of education and employment. For three decades the housing cost has gradually increased. Therefore, it translates that a sick person will not better their living standards. Instead, some become homeless while others find difficulties with the increasing cost of rent. The Little amount of money left after paying rent cannot cater for food, education and other necessities.

Inadequate housing put one at risk to become homeless, which in turn increases the likelihood of mental illnesses. Stress and depression occur not only to the parents, but also to children affecting their standard lifecycle. High incidence of homelessness increases violence, and such exposure increases fear, anxiety and stigmatization of poor people, thus making them vulnerable to mental disorders.

Housing problems among poor people introduce new challenges while pursuing work and education. Work remains vital in acquiring enough income to provide for the daily needs of a family. On the other hand, it also affects education where training offers a platform to understand the different mental illnesses, how to prevent them, and how to provide adequate treatment. Poverty causes poor housing, which in turn increases chances of psychological sickness (McWilliams, 2011).

People with mental disabilities are excluded from development programs. Primarily when growth projects are deliberated, people with

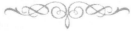

psychiatric disabilities are neither employed nor considered too much. Fewer chances of employment deprived them of their increase in income to solve mental health issues. It is contrary to the fact that different development project is meant to help and elevate the life of those most vulnerable in the society. Due to their high level of poverty, the mental illness can make them die prematurely.

Ways to Eradicate Poverty

The following methods can be employed when one seeks to eradicate poverty for those who are mentally ill.

First, there should be the administration of psychiatric drugs. Most of these drugs are used regularly, and some state governments offer them freely. Community-based rehabilitation facilities and programs must be conducted in areas where mental illness causes poverty or vice-versa. Family education about mental illness, its causes, treatment, and prevention come in handy to support the aim of existing institutions to reduce the occurrence of psychiatric disorders.

A conducive workplace environment for those who have mental illness must be adapted to reduce unnecessary pressure which may lead to resignation from work by these victims. Furthermore, human rights laws and policies must be fashioned to represent people with psychological and mental disabilities. The government, civil society, research institutes and other non-governmental institutions that champions the development agenda for vulnerable people should ensure poverty and mentally ill people are adequately considered for employment opportunities. Lastly, mental health education can be incorporated into the mainstream school to offer knowledge in dealing with mental illness.

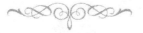

Summary, there is no way that one can speak about poverty and not mention mental illnesses. The two are entwined. Poor people face a lot of losses and encounter psychiatric diseases. These losses include credibility in workstations, their significant role on the society, lack of friends, and job loss due to their psychological state. Furthermore, their condition may be associated with lack of adequate housing facilities or a poor quality one, if they find family issues that revolve around stabilizing their mental conditions, physical health, trustworthiness in enjoyment and instances of low self-esteem. Everyone must take great care to avoid misinterpretation that given unlimited cash may help alleviate the mental illness. This is far from the truth, for only better medication, creating awareness and providing better living standard is helpful to those suffering individuals.

TREATMENT AND MENTAL HEALTH CARE IN THE BLACK COMMUNITY

A Brief history of Mental Health among the African American

Research conducted by the California Department of Mental Health indicates that the African American population suffers from mental health care and they do not receive proper treatment. Racism is one of the factors that affect the African American population when it comes to accessing mental health care. Culture bias prevails among African Americans due to the previous experiences of misdiagnosis. A census conducted in America during 1840-1930 concluded that blacks had a higher number of people suffering from mental health conditions. Another research conducted during 1940 to present, claims that during the selection of officers to go to the war many failed the test (Yasui, Hipwell, Stepp & Keenan, 2014). Majority of the men displayed psychiatric disorders. The research claims that the men who passed the test displayed different conditions known as acute psychiatric disorders. This paper will discuss the state of mental illness and treatment among African Americans.

Persistent and Emerging Issues in Mental Illness

Regardless of the research conducted by different scholars, the state of mental illness still needs to be addressed. The research to be conducted may help people understand the real state of the mental health issues at this time. The understanding of the cultural differences needs to be understood by the researchers before investigating on the state of mental health issues. The psychological and psychiatric status of blacks are two of the main

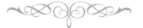

factors that need to be addressed before engaging in mental illness. Many African Americans are immigrants and the issue of identity contributes to stigmatization, thus psychological distress which results in mental illness (Godfrey et al., 2010).

The kind of life that African Americans live is one of the reasons why they are at a higher risk to suffer from mental health illness. The resources that they have are scarce, the environment where most of them live have high crime rates, poverty levels, and most of them do not have access to proper education. All these factors lead to psychological discomforts among those people. Racial segregation also has an influence in why African Americans receive few resources in their areas. The number of suicides committed by African Americans is higher than the whites. This is evidence to prove that the blacks are suffering from mental health illness and the problem needs to be addressed.

Misdiagnosis of Mental Health Illness

When accessing the racial differences between whites and blacks, it is notable that blacks do not receive proper mental health care treatment in comparison to whites. The resources allocated to their regions are not sufficient to provide necessary services. The other issue that arises when misdiagnosis of mental health illness is discussed among the African Americans is the culture. African Americans have a different perspective towards mental illness because of cultural influences. According to research, many have a tendency of treating any disorders that interfere with the normal functioning of the body.

Culture defines a way of life for people. Culture includes all the beliefs, practices and values that people have. According to the statistics provided

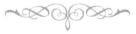

by the department of health in the US, most black women experience depression. According to Godfrey et al. (2010), black women do not receive proper health care during depression. This is a factor that will likely affect the black population because many African Americans have this belief of suffering alone and whenever someone has a problem, they believe that they will solve it on their own. Silence is assumed to be their treatment in such situations.

For depression to be properly treated, a patient must visit a psychologist to get the necessary help to overcome that condition. By following the traditional way of dealing with a problem, someone will end up suffering and eventually commit suicide which is the end-result of many cases of depression. A survey released by Wayne State University indicates that a large population of Americans received treatment for major depression, while African Americans had the lowest rate of seeking medical treatment for depression.

Treatment of Mental Health Problems
among African Americans

According to research conducted by various psychologists, African American people are more concerned with the stigma of the problem rather than focusing on the mental illness. Many African Americans prefer to deal with the problem on their own since they think that mental illness is not a condition that requires major medical attention. The following are some of the reasons why a large number of the black Americans do not address the issue of mental illness. The following subtopics will bring a clear picture of the state of treatment of mental illness among the black Americans.

Lack of Health Insurance

This is one of the reasons why African Americans do not seek medical treatment for their mental illness. Majority of African Americans do not have insurance coverage for medical care. The state of poverty among blacks encourages poor socioeconomic status, and further discourages them from acquiring medical insurance coverage (Godfrey et al., 2010).

The state of poverty among the African Americans is high and thus this problem, if not addressed, will worsen the mental health condition among African Americans. The National Poverty Center conducted research which clearly shows that there are high levels of poverty within the African American community. Most black women are single in the United States and single parenting is also one of the reasons why African American women suffer from mental illness. Poor mental health is due to the lack of funds to raise a child and many do not have enough resources to cover medical insurance. The following issues need to be addressed in order to move against the research that clearly states that less black Americans receive treatment for mental illness.

Shame and embarrassment

Among African Americans, mental health is a taboo subject to be discussed with anyone. Due to their beliefs, most black women do not seek treatment for any psychological disorder due to the shame and embarrassment that it can cause (Yasui, Hipwell, Stepp & Keenan, 2014). For the cases of mental health problems to begin to be diminished, many African Americans need to begin embracing change and acknowledge that most of the beliefs are obsolete.

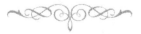

Lack of knowledge

The lack of knowledge among the African American community is an obstacle to accessing relevant authorities in cases of mental illness. Due to the myths and misconceptions surrounding the topic of mental illness, the African American population does not have adequate knowledge about the causes and the cure of such conditions. Majority of African Americans believe that the psychological disorders are just normal and thus the need for treatment is not a priority. The research conducted by the mental illness department in America, shows that there is a need to educate the black population in America on the causes of mental illness and the procedures that people need to go through to heal from those illnesses. The other challenge is trying to change the beliefs of African Americans concerning the topic of mental illness.

Lack of treatment

A large number of black women are undertreated when it comes to depression. A study conducted by the University of Wisconsin accounts for the reasons of undertreatment which include: gender discrimination, racism, and poverty (Yasui, Hipwell, Stepp & Keenan, 2014). The problem of lack of hospitals also prevailed in one of the studies conducted by the same university. African Americans do not receive proper mental health treatment, since there are few institutions to deal with such patients.

Refusal of help

As stated earlier, the state of mental health problems is worsening as many African Americans refuse to be treated appropriately. One of the

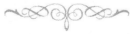

reasons that encourages them not to accept help is memories. They still remember what happened to them at the hands of white people. The issue of trust arises since many do not want to be helped by those who they claim made them go through misery during the time of slavery.

Under this subtopic, the other factor that makes African Americans not seek help in hospitals is because the quality of the health care provided is poor. The hospitals do not have competent psychiatrists who are able to treat them well. The other reason is that the majority of health care professionals in their area are not African American.

The extreme levels of cultural distrust among black Americans and white Americans are also a factor that makes black Americans not visit the hospital for proper mental health screening and care. In chapter 10, the focus will shift to discussing methods that can be put in place the eliminate mental health problems.

ELIMINATING HEALTH PROBLEMS
IN THE BLACK COMMUNITY

In this chapter, the discussion will shift to some of the methods that the government and the African American community can adopt to eliminate, or reduce the occurrence of mental health problems. The topics to be discussed below include education for the community, training more African American psychiatrist, change of beliefs, and infrastructure improvement.

Infrastructure Improvement

The government is supposed to ensure that people have opportunities to earn money, so that they can purchase proper medical insurance coverage. The American government should ensure that the poverty levels are decreased among the African American population. For single mothers, they can be given jobs that will help them to access medical health care. Another measure that the government can implement is partnering with other health organizations so that the provision of mental health therapy is free (Stansbury, Peterson & Beecher, 2013). The government should increase the number of doctors who are working at the mental institutions in such places. The treatment for mental illness is quite expensive. By either reducing or rendering free services, people will be freer to access the health care needed.

The number of institutions providing mental illness treatment are few. There is a need to construct more facilities to deal with mentally ill people at an affordable cost or even free, depending on the State's commitment on

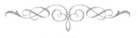

reducing the number of mentally ill patients. The trained and the competent psychiatrists should be deployed to such facilities so that they can provide quality healthcare to these patients.

Training More African American Psychiatrists

The African American clinicians should dominate the institutions which are constructed to provide treatment for African Americans. The deployment of the clinicians will increase the trust of the African Americans towards the health care institutions. This trust will enable African Americans to change their perspective and beliefs towards white Americans and will encourage living in cohesion (Stansbury, Peterson & Beecher, 2013).

Establishment of Acts, such as the Affordable Care Act, should be implemented so that more African Americans will continue registering for insurance coverage which will give them access to quality health care in different hospitals. The distribution of funds among the African American community should be sufficient to develop infrastructure such as hospitals, schools and other public facilities. The development of infrastructure will decrease the occurrences of depression among black Americans by enabling them to live a comfortable life. This is important since it is evident that some of the facilities, and the lack of suitable education causes depression in the young African Americans.

Racism and Change of Beliefs

Racism is also one of the factors that discourages African Americans from looking for medical attention when they see signs mental of illness. Many blacks have reported racial segregation in the hospitals and that

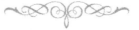

is why a small percentage visit the hospital with such problems. The therapists who are supposed to treat them end up mistreating them in the hospitals. The American Psychological Association is largely dominated by white Americans. Due to white domination, it is feared that the African American population does not know how to handle mental illness patients.

For the racists, their perspective toward their victims should change, since all humans are created equal. The only difference that is between them is color. By training more African Americans to be therapists, it will help the issue of racism to ease, since majority of the white Americans will come to realize that black Americans also have the same ability as them.

African Americans are mostly tied to their cultural beliefs. Some of the beliefs include that mental illness are caused by the aging process. Some of them believe that they do not need to consult a psychiatrist so that they can get help. They believe that their families will help them overcome such problems. Many African Americans lack knowledge to understand that mental cases need to be addressed by someone who is qualified, and can prescribe the appropriate treatment to address the issue. A qualified psychiatrist will be able to handle a patient well and help them to resume to their normal life after treatment. By implementing such rules, the number of mental illness cases will reduce. The country will be able to meet its goals of reducing the number of mental cases thus, increasing the human survival rate (Stansbury, Peterson & Beecher, 2013).

Shame and embarrassment is usually a common association that people with mental illness have with mental illness. The government has put in place programs which have educated African Americans about the issue of mental illness. The government has increased the number of African Americans who are psychiatrists. The training of the African American

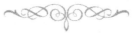

psychiatrists has been a success since it has helped the African American communities to gain knowledge about the problem of mental illness by one of their own. Black physiatrists have spread awareness on the need to stop stigmatizing the mentally ill patients, and encouraging people to take them to the proper facilities to be treated.

Through exposure to different cultures, African Americans can change their views towards the mental illness issue and can be influenced to seek medical treatment when necessary. Medical practitioners should try to engage the black community so that they interact with them to offer solutions to some of the mental cases, and advise them on the right procedure to use whenever someone is faced with a psychological problem. The government should also allocate enough funds to deal with mental illness since it is one of the major causes of suicides in America (Hays & Lincoln, 2017). By allocation of sufficient resources for the African American population, the government will ensure that there is proper use of money by educating the community about the causes of psychological disorders and how to deal with them. The programs formulated by the government to teach the community about mental health awareness will help decrease the stigma that comes along with mental illness. The people will then be more careful and vigilant if they show any signs of psychological problems.

African American history forces one to relive the evils done by white Americans and discourages them from accessing healthcare from these people. All this is caused by their negative attitude. For the African American population to be helped, a change of perspective is necessary in this area. The issue of racism should be highly condemned so that changes can be observed when it comes to the problem of mental illness.

Education Programs

African American leaders should create educational programs to create awareness to the community so that black Americans will be educated concerning the issues of mental illness. The community can be trained on how to deal with a mentally ill person and educate them on the channels that they will use in order that someone will get over their condition.

The community should also be educated on the causes of depression, and the signs and symptoms of mental illness. The facilitators should also encourage the African-Americans to attend the hospitals whenever they show any sign of mental illness. The education offered to the community will make them aware of the situations that will make them become less mentally ill. The purpose of the facilitators of the educational programs will be to educate the community on the dangers of mental illness, which includes: suicides, violence, and drug abuse.

Hays and Lincoln (2017), acknowledges that mental illness affects every 1 out of 5 Americans. The problem of mental illness needs to be addressed and not only to African American, citizens should be educated on how to manage mental illness, everyone should be educated. The educators should also encourage those with mental illnesses to visit hospitals and stick to the routines as advised by the therapists. The community will be aware of the condition of mental illness which will help in the decrease of mental illness case in America.

For the United States of America to be able to manage the rise of mental illness, campaigns should be done to try to identify those conditions as early as possible and begin early intervention.

Following these recommended methods will indeed have a great impact on the country by reducing the number of mental illness cases.

RACISM AS A MENTAL DISORDER

Ander, in (2012) acknowledges that racism has been the topic of discussion among Americans for many decades. The African American community has always been disregarded when compared to whites and has been denied equal access to resources. The historical experiences of blacks have a great influence on their mental health. Though the American Psychiatrists Association (APA) has made great progress in extending its services to the black community, blacks are still underrepresented and receive poor medical services in comparison to whites. The increased mental health problems among blacks can be attributed to the discrimination they continue to face in the western world based on their color. Whites are continuing to feel superior to blacks. They often regard blacks as weak and incapable of handling complex issues on their own. Their history, which displays them as a violent community, has also played a great role on the hostility that these people continue to face due to lack of trust from authorities.

Racism and Mental Health

Blacks have always been discriminated against and looked down upon by other races which consider themselves superior to blacks. One of the major revolutionaries in the field of exploring black discrimination is Dubois, who is of black descent. Dubois has written works which try to document racism and discrimination among the black community living in a country that is not originally theirs. Racism is viewed as the thought that one is superior to the other and is of detriment in their

culture. Discrimination is the negative way in which people treat others since the other group of people belong to a lower class.

Several theories have been used to show the relationship between racism and mental disorders. Those theories have been developed in Psychology and they have been used to show the procedure of treating and establishing racism related issues. Racism has been classified as a disease by psychologist. Those in the field of Biology tend to dispute that fact and classify racism as an issue to do with mental disorders.

A study conducted among 10,000 people have indicated that racism is strongly a mental disorder. Majority of the people who are said to be perpetrators of racism are said to have mental conditions such as: conduct disorder, depression, and defiant disorder among others (Mouzon & McLean, 2016).

African American individuals are usually segregated by other races. This may be one of the major causes of distress among those people. Distress is among the contributors to mental health. Other research, conducted by the national study of black Americans, indicates that the dissatisfaction and psychological stress among African-American people are the factors that affect the mental health of the black population.

Extreme racists are said to progress through five stages as described by Allport, which included verbal expression of antagonism, avoiding members of the minority group, active discrimination, physical attack, and then extermination. The signs of racism are visible which validates the argument that it is a mental disorder that can be treated. Once an individual begins to hate the other person based on race, he or she can make a point of seeking medical help by consulting a psychiatrist for professional counseling to help in solving the problem before it causes any

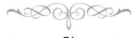

harm. Families should also help their relatives who are suffering from the same disorder. This can be done by helping them understand that it is an illness, and showing them the need to seek professional help.

The Dishonor of Inferiority and Mental Health

One of the psychological effects of racism is the harm that it causes to the affected victims who are diminished when it comes to their identity (Mouzon & McLean, 2016). The perpetrators of racism always attack the minority group making them feel superior and thus, creating distress among them. The discomfort caused by the attacks from the majority group causes the victim to develop stress which can progress to a more mature stage which is depression. Depression is among the symptoms of poor mental health.

The marginalized groups always have this belief that they are inferior to the other groups. This condition of inferiority encourages the stigmatized group to be affected both socially and psychologically. The effects of internalization are realized even when the two groups of people are taken to school. The marginalized group will perform poorly as compared to the highly regarded group. Internalized racism has made many blacks hate other people of their own kind and feel a discomfort around them. This is a factor which is a result of the usual inferiority complex.

The dishonor of racial inferiority may also make African American people receive under treatment or over treatment from the black psychiatrists due to the myths and misconceptions they have towards the blacks.

Health Consequences of Racism

Among the African American community, police are always on surveillance in those areas. The fact that police are around their homes in America is a cause of stress among those who live in those areas. When others have negative encounters with the police, their feelings may be aroused which causes psychological discomfort.

In the African American community, many children have witnessed people being shot dead by the police. Others have witnessed violence and that could affect their lives psychologically. Since the horrific scenes may not be erased from their minds, such kids may end up suffering from depression because they are always afraid of what will happen next. The horrendous scenes may even make them become violent when they grow up. The kids who are not strong enough to deal with such effects need to visit a psychiatrist, so that they can go through a therapy session and try to cope with those terrible murders and violent scenes.

High levels of crime among the African American community causes distress in lawbreakers and increases the number of fatalities. The aftermath of a death of a family member can create a psychological distress among those left behind, especially those who are still young.

Compound Dimensions of Racism

The highest number of criminal offenders are citizens of African American origin. A research carried out about the cause of death in America indicated that homicides were leading, and the black population is more vulnerable to homicides than the whites. The largest population of prisoners in America is African Americans (Anderson,

76

2012). The number of black people on probation is slightly higher than those of white people. This clearly indicates that black people are usually associated with criminal offenses in America.

One of the factors that make blacks commit a crime is the type of lives they live. Majority of the black people are poor, which forces them to engage in crime to pay their bills and eat. The state of joblessness also encourages blacks to commit crimes, contributing to 12% of people in prison as compared to 3% of white criminal offenders. In prison, research indicated that blacks receive more punishment than whites (Mouzon & McLean, 2016).

Crime affects the family members of the person who is arrested. The family members may suffer from poor mental health. The problem will adversely affect their attitude and their daily operations since there is a gap in their lives. Loneliness is a factor that can lead to depression, which will affect the normal functioning of someone's brain.

After someone is released from jail, they are likely to be affected by the new environment, because the criminal record that they possess may hinder them from getting jobs, since many firms do not hire people with criminal records. The firms are always afraid of a repetition of the same behavior. The criminal record also discourages people by making them feel like an outcast. Others may even decide to end their lives so that they will get out of this misery.

Conclusion

As indicated in many of the examples used in this chapter, racism is directly linked to mental health. African Americans are mostly the victims of racism in America as compared to other immigrants. There is a need

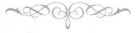

to disassemble the ideologies of racism so that the African American population can be saved from the mental health problems associated with racism.

The concept of racism should be analyzed carefully, and the health problems associated with it should be understood clearly. In our society today, racism is the basis of classifying people. Racism acts as a foundation for causes of health problems, but there are other factors that are responsible for poor mental health. A clear boundary should be established, and necessary courses of action should be taken towards saving the African American race. This could result in extinction, due to the number of mental illness cases that claim most people's lives within that community. The role of racism in mental health should be analyzed, and the ways in which racism changes people's health should to be established so that the perpetrators of racism can in some way be influenced to change their ways.

SUICIDE IN THE AFRICAN AMERICAN COMMUNITY

Suicide is the act of self-killing. It is all about self-slaughter, murder, destruction, and taking one's own life. The violence that is self-directed, which includes the suicidal behavior, is referred as an actual or threatened use of physical force against oneself, which leads to death or injury. Completed suicide or suicide is regarded as death from suffocation, poisoning, or harm where it is implicitly, or explicit evident that the damage was anticipated to be fatal and it was self-inflicted. In the United States, injury from suicidal was a leading public health problem. Among the young black men, suicide was a growing trend. In the black community, friends and family lived with undiagnosed depression which was going unnoticed, due to the stigma that was associated with mental health care. Black young children between the ages of 5-11 years had a shocking increase of suicide. As compared to the black children, white children had a lower suicidal rate of 1.96 which declined later to 1.31 %, unlike the black children whose rate increased from 1.96% to 3.47%.

Due to the higher rate of suicide cases among African American people, the emotional and social support such as community connectedness, Peer and Family support were established to assist in protecting black adolescents from their behavior of committing suicide. Likewise, the family and social support and positive interactions were developed to reduce the suicidal risk amongst black adults (Hirsch, et al, 2014). Among religions, personal devotion and Orthodox religious beliefs were identified to protect blacks against suicide. Nevertheless the organized spiritual participation practices

like attending the church had a lower rate of committing suicide among African Americans. Religiosity was found to be of higher importance for blacks who had psychiatric disorders as it delayed the ideation age of onset, hence reducing the mental disorders.

African Americans had a lower rate of suicide attempts as compared to the Caribbean Blacks. African American black adolescent males' rate was higher than those of Caribbean Blacks. Even though when comparing the U.S. overall suicide rates, the blacks had a lower rate, but on the side of the youth, it had the rate that was higher than that of the adults. Suicide was third among the leading cause of deaths in the black kids. In that case, the number of deaths has a more significant impact on the black community at large. For the blacks of all ages, suicide was the 16th, and for the male youth, it was the 3rd cause of death. To attempt suicide, females are more likely to attempt while males are more likely to complete.

For several reasons, it is hard when talking about suicide. Not only that blacks are turning their backs from the reality of suicide in their communities, but they are always combating the mental health stigma. It is in rare cases people can hear the impact that suicide has on their family members and friends or about those who lost their lives in such manner. Self-murder has a way of producing a trail of isolation, shame, sadness, and guilt which perpetuates further stigma. Many people believe that blacks do not kill themselves, but that is a myth. To say the truth is that many had been impacted by suicide in one way or the other. It was a culture for the black to pretend that suicide is a weakness and they cannot take it, and it was only their relationship with God should shield them on the pains they can't handle (Brockie, et al., 2015) They assume that black people do not die from suicide as a way of forgetting

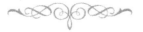

the pain of losing their loved loves. The reality is that, these are some circumstances or factors that put individuals at risk for suicide, like exposure to racial oppression and inequality, skills of maladaptive coping, family dysfunction, exposure to violence, homelessness, social isolation, access to firearms and weapons, substance abuse, and psychological distress. Black communities are at the suicidal risk because distrust and stigma of mental health professionals, inadequate insurance coverage of mental health, and proximity to services and access to mental health services are limited.

Apart from healthcare gaps and police brutality, numerous types of systemic violence have affected the black communities. But mental health stigma which is an overlooked threat has a deadly effect on black children. For blackness to be synonymous with pain such notion needs to be combated by knowing that black people also need to live with joy, regardless of race. Although white people have a higher number of suicide rates in the country, for black children, it is increasing by the day. Such sudden increase has shown how the population of black children has been chipped away quietly by mental health problems. It is hard for blacks to do away with mental health, because once affected, it remains stigmatized profoundly, unlike for white people. Due to mistrust, the stigmatized people need to be around someone whom they feel safe, someone who has a sense of understanding their pressure and what they are going through in life. For this reason, Archbold notes that for the blacks to feel more comfortable, the number of social workers and black doctors need to be increased. Such is the only way that will make the black community accept health care by trusting their doctors. For black people, it is not easy to believe the health professionals, as there was medical experts' history of violating their trust.

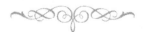

Hence, many families rely on spiritual healing rather than going to the medical professional.

Consequently, such distrust among medical professionals could leave children with severe mental health untreated or undiagnosed resulting in long-term neglect. In that regard, mental health screenings should be set in predominant churches of the blacks to enable them to approach individuals in a comfortable space. Black people should combat the notion that blackness is synonymous with pain by overcoming trauma even though it is not so simple. Archbold is an excellent example of a black lady who battled quietly with suicidal thoughts in her teenage years and embraced the label she was hesitant. For black people, being too proud to accept help is the strength which means carrying a heavy load of suffering and stress silently. For the black girls, it was an unrealistic stereotype, but Archbold faced her weaknesses and found her strength. And many black girls went through the same struggle. In a black community, the weakness of emotion was looked down upon. It is time for the black people to shift the stigma which was ignored for a long time by embodying themselves to seek for care by using their pride of endurance. Such strength should open the way for easy access to mental health resources by black people.

Thus, it is time for black people to redefine what we want, and stop being blinded by pride while suffering. It is time for the blacks to move out of suicides by swallowing their pride and seek the care of the health centers and rehabilitation homes. Such a step will enable them to move out of depression, stress, and silent suffering that triggers an individual towards having a suicidal mind as a solution to their problems. The black community needs to stand on their own and say no to suicides, say no to save their families, and say no to save their friends from such problems by

opposing the notion of blackness is synonymous. They should know that they were not born to suffer; rather to enjoy life by kicking out blackness as a compatible notion.

Black people should seek assistance from the emotional and social support such as community connectedness, Peer and Family support which was established to assist in protecting the Black adolescents from their behavior of committing suicide. Likewise, the family and social support and positive interactions were developed to reduce the suicidal risk among black adults. Thus, that is how self-murder impacts the black community at large.

REFERENCES

Alegria. M., Canino, G., R., Vera, M., Calderon, J., Rusch, D., & Ortega. A.N. (2012). Mental health care for Latinos: Inequalities in use of specialty mental health services among Latinos, African Americans, and non-Latino Whites. Psychiatric Services, 53(12), 1547-1555.

Anderson, K. (2012). Diagnosing Discrimination: Stress from Perceived Racism and the Mental and Physical Health Effects*. Sociological Inquiry, 83(1), 55-81. http://dx.doi.org/1 0. I I 1 1/j.1475-682x.2012.00433.x

Brockie, T. N., Dana-Sacco, G., Wallen, G.R., Wilcox, H.C., & Campbell, J.C. (2015). The Relationship of Adverse Childhood Experiences to PTSD, Depression, Poly-Drug Use and Suicide Attempt in Reservation-Based Native American Adolescents and Young Adults. American journal of community psychology, 55(3-4), 411-421.

Cartwright S. Diseases and peculiarities of the Negro race. 1851. Available at: Htt://www.pbs.org/wgbh/aia/part4/4h3 1 06t.hbnl. Accessed November 1, 2017.

Connolly, Adrian J. (2008). "Personality disorders in homeless drop-in center clients" (PDF). Journal of Personality Disorders. 22 (6): 573-588.

Erlanger A. Turner, P. (2017, June 27). *#YouGoodMan: Black Men and Mental Health.* Journal of Personality Disorders. 22 (6): 573-588.

Erlanger A. Turner, P. (2017, June 27). *#YouGoodMan: Black Men and Mental Health.* Retrieved from https://m.huffpost.com/us/entry/us 5951 de6ae4b0c85b96c65c3d

Geller A.F. (2014). Aggressive policing and the mental health of young urban men. *American Journal of Public Health,* 104 (12), 2121-2127.

Godfrey, E., Yoshikawa. H., Jost. J., Aber, J., Hughes, D., & Suarez-Orozco, C. (2010). *Motive vs. status: System justification, mental health andproblem behavior among immigrant and ethnically diverse mothers and their children.*

Hays, K., & Lincoln, K. (2017). Mental Health Help-Seeking Profiles Among African Americans: Exploring the Influence of Religion. *Race and Social Problems,* 9(2), 127-138. http//dx.doi.org/10.1007/s12552-01 7-9193-1

Hirsch, J.K., Nsamenang, S. A., Chang, E., & Kaslow, N.J. (2014). Spiritual weJl-being and depressive symptoms in female African American suicide attempters: Mediating effects of optimism and pessimism. Psychology of Religion and Spirituality, 6(4), 276.

Logan, S., Denby, R., & Gibson, P.A. (Eds.). 2013. *Mental health care in the African-American Community. Routledge.*

Mata. D. A.; Ramos, M.A.; Bansal, N; Khan, R; Guille, C; Di Angelantonio, E; Sen, S (2015). "Prevalence of Depression and Depressive Symptoms Among Resident Physicians: A Systematic Review and Meta-analysis". JAMA. 314 (22): 2373-2383.

Matthew & Hughes TL. (2001). Mental health service use by African American women: Exploration of subpopulation differences. *Cultural Diversity and Ethnic Minority Psychology 7(1), 75-87.*

McWilliams, Nancy (2011). Psychoanalytic Diagnosis: Understanding Personality Structure in the Clinical Process (200 ed.). Guilford Press. ISBN 978-1-60918-494-0

Mouzon, D., & McLean, J. (2016). Internalized racism and mental health among African-Americans, US-born Caribbean Blacks, and foreign-born Caribbean Blacks. *Ethnicity & Health,* 22(1), 36-48. http://dx.doi.org{I 0.1080/13557858.2016.1196652

Oakley LD, S.M.-M. (2005). Positive and negative depression coping in low-income African American women. *Research in Nursing 2,* 106-116.

Russon, John (2003). Human Experience: Philosophy, Neurosis, and the Elements of Everyday Life. State University ofNew York Press. ISBN 0-7914-5754-0

Schnittker, J., Freese, J., & Powell, B. (2013). Nature, neither, nor: Black-White differences in beliefs about the causes and appropriate treatment of mental illness. *Social Forces,* 78(3), 1101-1132.

Stansbury, K., Peterson, T., & Beecher, T., & Beecher, B. (2013). An exploration of mental health literacy among older African Americans. *Aging & Mental Health, 17*(2), 226-232. http://dx.doi.org/1 0.1080/ 1 3607863.2012. 724652

Swartz, M.S., Swanson, J. W., Hiday, V. A., Borum, R., Wagner, H.R., & Burns, B.J. (2015). Violence and severe mental illness: the effects of substance abuse and non-adherence to medication. *Americanjournal ofpsychiatry, 155(2), 226-231.*

Ward, E.C., Wiltshire, J.C., Detry, M.A., & Brown, R.L. (2013). African American men and women's attitude toward mental illness, perceptions of stigma, and preferred coping behaviors. *Nursing Research,* 62(3), 185-194. Doi:10.1097/NNR. Ob013e31827b:f533

Whaley AL. (200 I). Cultural mistrust of white mental health clinicians among African Americans with severe mental illness. *American Journal of Orthopsychiatry 71 (2), 252-256.*

Williams, M.T. (2013). How therapists drive away minority clients. Psychology Today. Retrieved from https://www.psychologytoday.com/blog/culturally -speaking/201306/ how-therapists-drive•away-minority-c...

Yasui, M., Hipwell, A., Stepp, S., & Keenan, K. (2014). Psych cultural Correlates of Mental Health Service Utilization Among African American and European American Girls. *Administration and*

Policy in Mental Health and Mental Health Services Research, 42(6), 756-766. http://dx.doi.org/ IO. I 007/s 10488-014-0610-0

Young, J.L., Griffith, E., & Williams, D.R. (2013). The integral role of pastoral counseling by African-American clergy in community mental health. *Psychiatric Services. 54(5). 688-692.*

CPSIA information can be obtained
at www.ICGtesting.com
Printed in the USA
LVHW09s2134140818
586849LV00004BA/326/P